JUICING 101

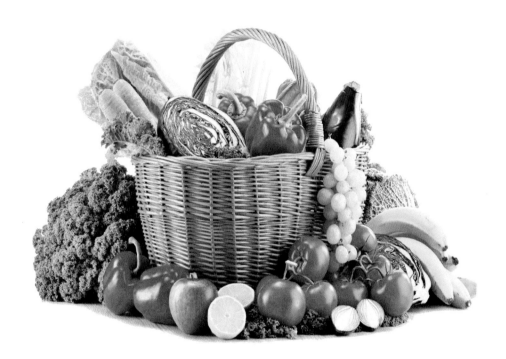

ZAIRE PUBLISHING

NOTICE

Library of Congress Cataloging-in-Publication Data

Leffall, Harold

Juicing 101: The Essential Guide to Good Health and Weight Loss

Table Of Contents

Introduction

"A recent study was conducted that evaluated surveys of 500 people on a living foods diet; the study revealed amazing health benefits from choosing raw foods such as freshly made juice that is the supreme raw food. The research showed that more than 80 percent of the individuals who participated in the survey, lost weight. But that was only the commencement of their transformation phase."

-Cherie Calbom, America's Most Trusted Nutritionist

In a world full of fad diets, it is challenging to unveil the most effective weight loss plan that delivers the best health with the benefits of a healthy weight loss. When looking for an effective weight loss program, you might consider a low-calorie diet with the biggest share of nutrients to keep your body healthy during the process.

To cater to all your needs, Juicing is the ultimate body detoxifier that lowers your calories to shed off all your excess fat while preventing the development of any life-threatening disorder. It provides the body with all the necessary vitamins, minerals, fibers, antioxidants, and a boost of energy without the use of caffeinated beverages.

The so-called "Western American Diet" has diverged into a diet that mainly consists of foods containing little to no fiber and high amounts of processed carbohydrates, proteins, saturated fats, and sugars. All these components, if consumed in an excessive amount, can eventually lead to life-threatening conditions. Some major health risks correlated with poor dietary and nutritional practices are Type II Diabetes, hypertension, cardiovascular disorders, various forms of cancer, and stroke.

To avoid such health dilemmas, one must be willing to let go of their unhealthy food habits and start consuming a well-balanced diet abundant in disease-preventing foods. Such foods may include fresh fruits and raw vegetables that are high in antioxidants and play a dominant role in defending the body against harmful chemicals.

Scientific research supports the idea of fresh Juicing and raves about its numerous health benefits, including weight loss, better digestion, stronger immunity, the capacity to fight allergies and infections, relief women's health problems, and a sound and peaceful sleep. Many medical journals have conducted studies that have acknowledged the benefits of specific juices and their role in the prevention of certain health conditions.

My Healing Journey

Like many others, my health awakening journey took its earliest steps in 2015 when I was at the age of 48 and was diagnosed with prostate cancer. I was extremely shocked and devastated because earlier that year, I witnessed the death of two of my younger friends due to cancer, but I never thought that cancer would find its way to my door. In my opinion, my health rituals were good enough to keep me healthy and safe; I exercised regularly, maintained a healthy weight, and did not consume a lot of red meat.

Later on, after I was diagnosed with cancer, I began to research the root cause of this illness, and I was surprised to learn that there were many strings attached to the things that I consumed on a regular basis to cancer.

Scientific evidence proved that the consumption of diet sodas, high-fat dairy products (consisting of cheese that I love a lot), fried foods, processed meat, and added sugars, and even microwaved popcorn, all contained cancer-causing agents.

I was so overwhelmed about why I wasn't aware of all of this? We all grew up hearing that milk provides healthy nutrients to the body, but we didn't realize that the fat in milk may lead to something serious. All this misinformation led to my quest to study more about health and nutrition to heal myself and others.

According to David Eisenberg, adjunct associate professor at Harvard T.H. Chan School of Public Health told NewsHour,

"Despite the connection between poor diet and many preventable diseases, only about one-fifth of American medical schools require students to take a nutrition course. Today, most medical schools in the United States teach less than 25 hours of nutrition courses for over four years. The fact that less than 20 percent of medical schools have a single required course in nutrition is a scandal. It's outrageous, and it's obscene!"

I was astounded that doctors receive little to no education on the association of nutrition to healthcare in medical schools. To some extent, it makes sense because doctors are obliged to simply hand over a prescription for the ailment rather than addressing the root cause and treat it with all the potential methods that incorporate nutrition.

Over the course of 5 years since my cancer diagnosis, I have been endeavoring to study and explore all the conceivable approaches to fuel my body and provide appropriate nutrition to treat my sickness.

Since that day, Juicing has been my ultimate reality and a fundamental part of my healing journey. Today at the age of 53, I am at the peak of my health, and to be honest, I have never been this healthy ever before! I have a cancer-free life, an ideal weight, clear skin, improved sleep, and enhanced cognition, and many more to be counted.

To benefit others to fight this deadly disease like me, who have been grieving cancer or other health-related problems, I came up with a solution to put together all of my secrets into one place and provide it to others to share a healthy life with me.

In Juicing 101: The Essential Guide to Good Health and Weight Loss, I present you with all the real strategies that I have adopted to lose weight, live better, feel better, and look better.

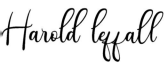

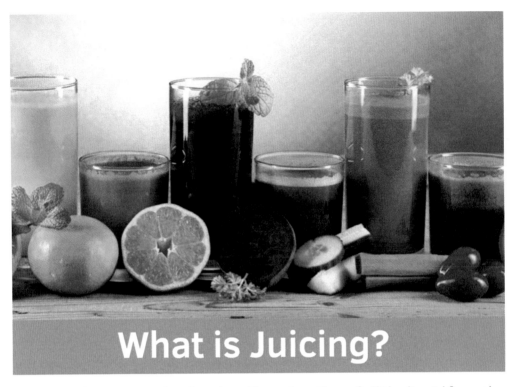

What is Juicing?

Juicing is the process that involves the extraction of all the liquid from the pulp of fruits or vegetables. Fresh juice consists of the same nutrients that an original fruit and vegetable contain. Juicing is an efficient and effortless approach to meet your daily quota for all essential vitamins, minerals, carotenes, and other valuable cancer-fighting agents. The idea of juicing is not very widespread, but people are digging deeper into the world of juicing due to its ravishing benefits and an incredible assortment. Either if you are seeking to add a glow to your skin or to fight the deadliest of diseases, i.e., cancer, juicing with its wide variety will present the best recipes to fulfill all your desires of living a healthy and fit life. Let's dive into some excellent gains of juicing!

Health Benefits of Juicing:

Acts as Stress-Reducers:

An article published by Shannon Wongvibulsin, a BS Candidate at UCLA in the year 2014, stated, "Proper diet can counterbalance the influence of stress by strengthening the immune system, stabilizing moods, and reducing blood pressure."

Fruits and vegetables are rich in vitamins, especially vitamin C, which significantly reduces the levels of cortisol in your body. Cortisol is the hormone that induces stress, and due to the lowering of this hormone, stress levels may instantly drop while providing you a life free of depression, anxiety, and tension.

Berries, oranges, kale, broccoli, grapefruit, guava, and papaya, and many more fruits and veggies are high in vitamin C that aids to tackle stress.

The Best Defender Against Ailments:

The best defense against any virus or disease is a robust immune system, and to attain a healthy immune system, it is vital to keep your nutrient intake complete. Juicing plays a massive role in building your immunity as it delivers the daily share of nutrients and antioxidants that fights against infections and viruses and also prevents the development of life-threatening disorders.

Blood Pressure Regulator:

Fluctuating blood pressure patterns may affect your health and well-being and cause an emotional imbalance that makes it challenging to execute daily life activities. Juicing is the best method to lower your raised blood pressure while promoting a healthy weight loss. The blood pressure-lowering impact of raw foods is most likely due to healthier food choices consisting of the right amounts of fiber and potassium.

A book named The Complete Book of Juicing, written by Michael Murray in 1992, says, if you carefully look at the human body system, you will find that humans need more potassium in their diets for the maintenance of normal blood pressure. But, the majority of obese Americans consume more sodium in their foods rather than potassium. Higher amounts of sodium and lower potassium levels can make your body fall prey to greater health risks and eventually lead to the development of cancer and cardiovascular diseases.

The Ultimate Body Detoxifier:

Once you start the juicing diet, you will begin to consume high-quality meals that contain all the essential and non-essential nutrients. It will help eliminate toxins from your body and initiate the formation of newer, healthier cells and tissues.

For example, once you limit or stop taking your daily energizers such as tea, coffee, or chocolate, headache and migraines may start taking away your energy, forcing you to shut down all your activities. The pains are the body's general cleansing mechanism or regeneration process. Your brilliant and smart body discards the toxins like caffeine or theobromine from your body tissues and transports them out of the body via your bloodstream.

Similarly, the liver and kidneys overwork to discard the toxins from the blood because these temporarily increased toxin levels may provoke side effects such as headache, joint pain, or weakening of a limb. You may also experience a slower and heavier heart rate, which your mind may translate as lethargy, or lower energy levels.

Drinking Juice Before Sleeping:

If you yearn for a peaceful slumber, this nighttime beverage can help you win the calmest sleep of your life. Among the unlimited variety of juices, cherry juice is well-known for its high melatonin levels that induce a deep sleep stage. Additionally, drinking grape juice at night can also burn your calories while you are wandering in the beautiful valleys of your sleep. Research recommends that drinking a small glass of grape juice before falling asleep will help to cause insulin secretion at night that regulates the circadian rhythm and offers a sound slumber.

The Secret to Clear and Glowing Skin:

Juicing helps to detoxify the body from all the unwanted toxins and harmful chemicals that may cause any skin reaction, ranging from acne to anti-aging. It provides all the vitamins and minerals that your body requires to maintain a healthy glow on your skin. Nutrition is highly related to skin, hair, and nails; hence a good diet has always been essential for the maintenance of your inner and outer health.

Research suggests that vitamins, carotenoids, tocopherols, flavonoids, and a diversity of plant extracts have been proclaimed to possess potent antioxidant properties. All these have been extensively used in the skincare and makeup productions either as topical agents or as oral supplements to prolong youthful skin appearance.

BLENDING VS JUICING

The difference between blending and juicing... when you blend, the whole of the fruit or vegetable including the pulp (fiber) goes into the drink. Body energy and enzymes are expended when digesting the pulp. Consequently, it takes more effort for nutrients to be absorbed and less nutrients are being assimilated. This means healing is slower, compared to juicing.

Juicing on the other hand removes the tough fiber, making the resultant drink quicker and easier for the body to absorb.

_____

HEALTH BENEFITS
OF FRUITS

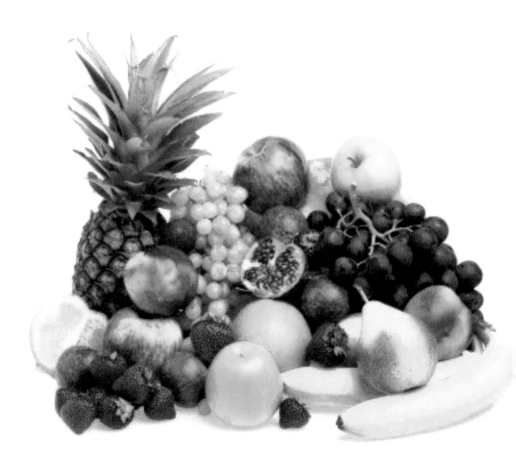

Apple: Contain antioxidants, vitamin C, fiber, and several other nutrients that may boost heart, brain, and digestive health.

Avocado: Contains vitamin B6 and folic acid, which help regulate homocysteine levels. High level of homocysteine is associated with an increased risk of heart disease.

Banana: Are rich in B vitamins, which help promote healthy sleep patterns and reduce irritability. Bananas also have vitamin C in addition to potassium and magnesium, all of which help to replenish the body's store of electrolytes.

Blackberry: Are low in calories and high in nutrition and support bone health. They are a rich source of vitamin C, vitamin K1 and manganese.

Blueberry: Contain pectin as well as flavonoids, which may help reduce your risk for type 2 diabetes. They are also rich in vitamin C, potassium, and tannins, which have antiviral and antibacterial properties. Additionally, blueberries contain manganese, which contributes to healthy bone growth.

Cantaloupe: Is an excellent source of folic acid, beta-carotene, fiber, potassium, and vitamin C.

Cranberry: Are rich in antioxidants and phytochemicals that promote a healthy immune system. Cranberries are also helpful for urinary tract issues and kidney stones.

Grape: Contain powerful antioxidants known as polyphenols. They also contain flavonoids, a powerful antioxidant that can help repair damage caused by free radicals – this property makes grapes an excellent anti-aging aid.

Grapefruit: Is an excellent source of vitamin C and is known as a natural fat burner.

Kiwi: Is an excellent source of vitamin C. It also contains vitamin K, vitamin E, folate, copper, and potassium. The enzymes found in kiwi have been shown to soothe stomach issues and may reduce the appearance of wrinkles.

Lemon: Rich in calcium, magnesium, potassium, and phosphorus. It is often referred to as the most powerful fruit for detoxification. It has been linked to cancer prevention, reduced heart disease and stroke.

Lime: Are a good source of magnesium and potassium, which promote heart health. Potassium can naturally lower blood pressure and improve blood circulation, which reduces your risk of a heart attack and stroke.

Mango: Rich in pre-biotic dietary fiber, vitamins, minerals, and poly-phenolic flavonoid antioxidant compounds. According to new research study, mango fruit has been found to protect from colon, breast, leukemia, and prostate cancers.

Melon: Contain a high content of carotenoids that can prevent cancer and lower the risk of lung cancer.

Orange: Contain D-limonene which has been shown to be effective in the prevention of cancers like breast cancer, colon cancer, lung cancer, and skin cancer. Vitamin C in oranges also acts as an antioxidant that protects cells from damages by free radicals.

Papaya: Is rich in antioxidants, such as lycopene, that may defend against the visible signs of aging.

Passion Fruit: Contains a high amount of vitamin A and vitamin C, both are strong antioxidant. They neutralize free radicals and protect from cancer.

Peach: Contains boron, niacin, and vitamin B3 which has been shown to reduce the risk of cardiovascular disease. Also, an excellent source of vitamin A and potassium.

Pear: A rich source of important minerals, such as copper and potassium. Copper plays a role in immunity, cholesterol metabolism, and nerve function, whereas potassium aids muscle contractions and heart function.

Pineapple: Contain trace amounts of vitamins A and K, phosphorus, zinc, and calcium. Rich in vitamin C and manganese. Manganese is a naturally occurring mineral that aids growth, maintains a healthy metabolism, and has antioxidant properties.

Pomegranate: Contain punicalagins and punicic acid, unique substances that are responsible for most of their health benefits. Pomegranates have potent anti-inflammatory properties, which are largely mediated by the antioxidant properties of the punicalagins which has been shown to lower blood pressure levels in as little as two weeks.

Raspberry: Have a high concentration of ellagic acid, a phenolic compound that helps lower the risk of cancer.

Strawberry: Have anti-inflammatory properties, which help with muscular pains and bone diseases.

HEALTH BENEFITS OF VEGETABLES

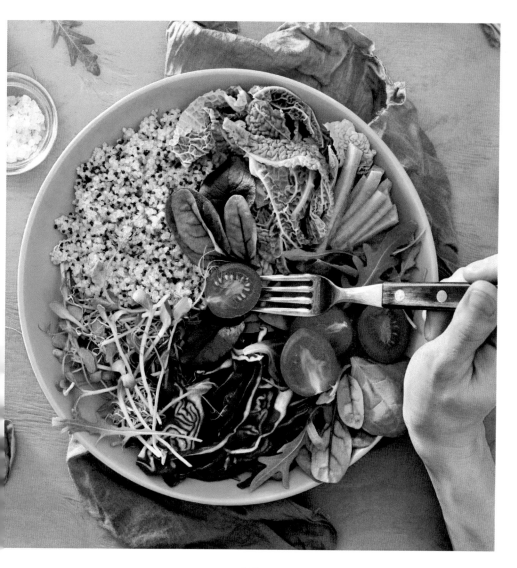

Beet: An excellent source of iron, choline, iodine, manganese, potassium, and vitamins A and C. Beets help to oxygenate the blood.

Bell Pepper: Contain high levels of vitamin C, which is essential for healing wounds and for maintaining eye and gum health. Also contains vitamin A, which is a key contributor to skin and eye health.

Bok Choy: Contains a variety of phytonutrients, vitamins, and minerals. It is also a good source of antioxidants.

Cabbage: Contains vitamin E and is rich in sulfur, which has been shown to help purify the blood and detoxify the liver. It also contains antibacterial, antioxidant, and anti-inflammatory properties.

Carrot: A great source of vitamins A, B, and C as well as iron, calcium, potassium, and sodium. Carrots also contain beta-carotene and carotenoid, which help reduce the risk for cancer, cardiovascular disease, and macular degeneration.

Cauliflower: Is high in B vitamins, phosphorus, potassium, manganese, and vitamin K. It is also a good source of antioxidants as well as glucosinolates, which help support the liver's detox abilities.

Celery: Is rich in a variety of vitamins and minerals. The silicon content of celery helps to strengthen joints and bones. It has also been shown to have diuretic and anti-cancer properties.

Cucumber: Great source of potassium and phytosterols, which help to lower cholesterol. Also, a good source of B vitamins and may help control blood pressure.

Garlic: Is known for its antimicrobial, antibiotic, and anti-cancer properties. It helps to lower blood cholesterol levels and blood sugar.

Ginger: Is great for detoxing as it cleanses the body and helps to support healthy digestion. It also has anti-nausea, anti-inflammatory, and antioxidant properties.

Kale: Is the highest vegetable source of vitamin K, which may help reduce the risk of certain cancers. It is a great source of calcium, iron, and chlorophyll.

Mint: A good source of plant-based omega-3 fatty acids, which support healthy hair, skin, and nails. It also helps with indigestion and inflammation.

Pumpkin: Is high in vitamins C and E as well as copper, iron, and potassium. Pumpkins has been shown to reduce risk of prostate cancer.

Spinach: Is a great source of calcium, iron, potassium, and protein. The iron content helps to build healthy blood cells.

Sweet Potato: Is high in copper, iron, magnesium, manganese, and other nutrients. It is beneficial for eye health, detoxification, digestive support and have anti-cancer properties.

Tomato: Is a good source of vitamin C, potassium, copper, iron, and magnesium. They have over nine thousand phytonutrients, including the antioxidant lycopene, which has been linked to cancer prevention.

Zucchini: Is a good source of copper, iron, magnesium, manganese, phosphorus, potassium, and vitamin C. It is also a good source of niacin (vitamin B3), which has been linked to reduced risk for cardiovascular disease.

According to the Dietary Guidelines for Americans, eating between five and 13 servings of veggies and fruit daily is ideal for good health. These total recommended serving amounts equal between 2 ½ to 6 1/2 cups of fruits and vegetables each day, depending on the number of calories you consume based on your weight and activity level.

PLANT PROTEIN

Protein helps keep the body healthy by building and repairing body tissues, coordinating with bodily functions, and allowing metabolic functions to take place. A diet that is high in plant protein is also linked to a reduced risk of diabetes, obesity, and heart disease.

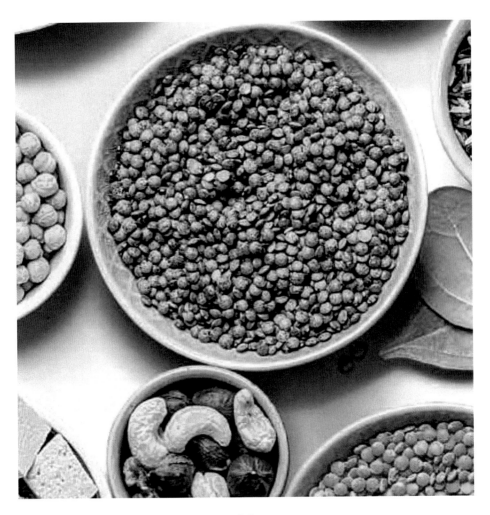

Asparagus

A cup of asparagus contains 2.95 grams of protein.

Broccoli

One stalk of broccoli, which is around 151 grams, contains approximately 4.26 grams of protein.

Cauliflower

Contains 2.05 grams of total protein per cup serving.

Kale

Contains 2.92 grams of protein per 100-gram serving.

Mushrooms

A cup of mushroom contains around 2.97 grams of protein.

Peas

A cup of frozen or edible-podded peas contains around 4.03 grams of protein.

Spinach

One package of spinach, which is around 284 grams, contains 8.12 grams of protein.

Generally, men need approximately 50-60 grams of protein daily, while women need around 40-45 grams of protein.

CHOOSING A JUICER

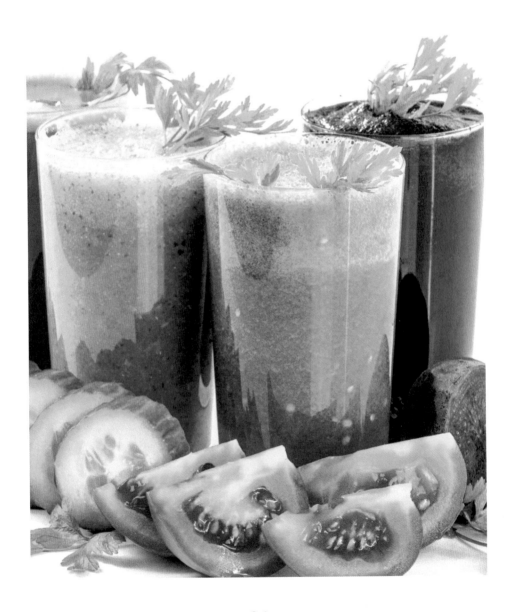

Centrifugal Juicers

A centrifugal juicer is the simplest type of juicer on the market. It is easy to clean and easy to operate. These juicers work fast and offer the most affordable options. On the downside, these juicers tend to be louder and the high-speed spinning causes the juice to oxidize faster than it would with slower speed juicers. As a result, it is best to drink juices from a centrifugal juicer the same day to ensure you receive the most nutrients.

Popular choices for centrifugal juicers: Breville Juice Fountain Compact, Omega, and Cuisinart Juice Extractor. A more affordable brand options include the juicers by Hamilton Beach and Jack LaLanne.

Masticating Juicers (AKA Slow Juicers)

A masticating juicer operates more slowly than a centrifugal juicer. These juicers operate like teeth – they use a single gear (or auger) that chews up your produce in order to break down the fibrous cell walls and extract the juice, which is gently squeezed through a stainless steel screen. Masticating juicers tend to yield more juice than centrifugal juicers, and therefore dryer pulp. Because they run at slower speeds, you get less oxidation and more nutrients. Plus, the juice last longer. You can store juices for up to 48 hours in a tightly sealed mason jar and refrigerate. These juicers are noticeably quiet.

Popular choices for masticating juicers: Hurom Slow Juicer, Omega Nutrition System Juicer, Omega VRT350, Breville Fountain Crush Slow Juicer, and the Champion Household Juicer.

Twin Gear Juicers (AKA Triturating Juicers)

A trituration juicer is a twin-gear juicer that utilizes a two-step juicing process. Twin gear juicers operate at even slower speeds than masticating juicers, which means it extracts the most juice and retain the highest nutrients. Because there is less oxidation, you can store your juice for up to 72 hours in an airtight glass container and refrigerate. Also, it is good for juicing wheatgrass. On the downside, the prep time involves cutting the produce into smaller sizes because the mouth of the machines is typically narrow. Feeding the juicer takes time because the gears turn slowly.

These juicers are more expensive and are the go-to choice for health gurus.

Popular choices for twin gear juicers: Super Angel 5500, Samson Green Power, Green Star Elite Juicer Extractor.

FRUIT BASED JUICES

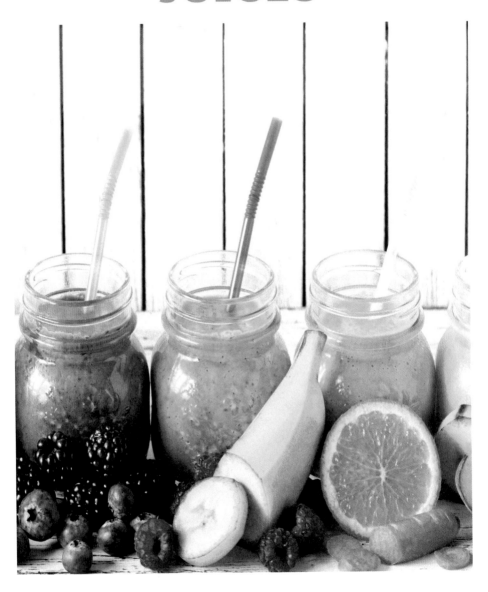

PINEAPPLE BLAST

Apple (1 large)

Pineapple (2 cups)

Pears (3 medium)

Ginger (1/2 thump tip)

Mint (1/4 cup)

Serve: 2

CRANBERRY DELIGHT

Apples (2 medium)

Orange (2 medium)

Cranberry (2 cups)

Pomegranate 1 cup)

Cilantro (6 sprigs)

Serve: 2

ORANGE ENERGY

Orange (2 medium)
Pineapples (3 cups)
Ginger (2 thumb tip)
Serve: 1

PINK PANTHER

Pomegranate (1 large)
Apple (1 large)
Orange (1 large)
Lemon (1 medium)
Ginger Root (1/2 thumb tip)
Serve: 1

PEACH DELIGHT

Apples (2 medium)
Peaches (2 medium)
Orange (1 medium, peeled)
Raspberry (1 cup)
Sparking Water (4 fl oz)
Lemon (1/2, peeled)
Serve: 2

STRAWBERRY BLITZ

Apples (1 medium)
Watermelon (1 cup, diced)
Strawberry (1 cup, whole)
Orange (1 medium)
Serve: 1

SUMMER VIBES

Pomegranate (1 cup)

Blueberry (1 cup)

Lemon (1 small)

Serve: 1

ORANGE THERAPY

Carrots (14 medium)

Apples (2 medium)

Orange (1 large, peeled)

Serve: 2

VEGETABLE BASED JUICES

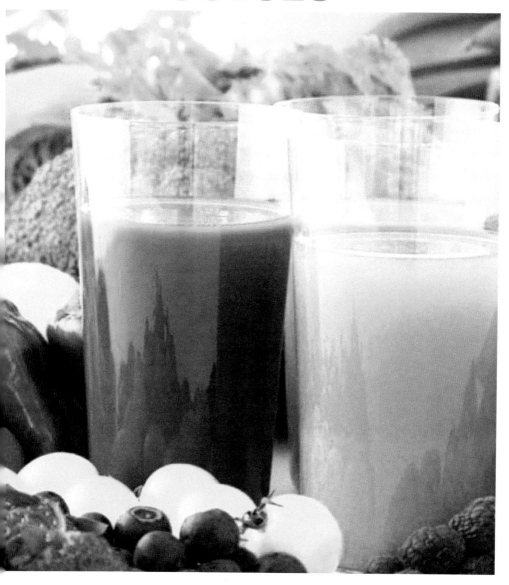

GINGER LEMONADE

Wheatgrass (1 bunch)

Lemon (1 large)

Apples (4 medium)

Carrots (2 medium)

Ginger (2 thumb tip)

Serve: 2

CRANBERRY CLEANSER

Pear (1 medium)

Apple (1 medium)

Cucumber (1 medium)

Celery (1 stalk, large)

Spinach (handful)

Cranberries (1/2 cup)

Serve: 1

GREEN GOODNESS

Apples (3 medium)

Celery (4 stalks, large)

Orange (1 large, peeled)

Spinach (5 handful)

Lemon (1/2)

Ginger Root (1/2 thumb tip)

Serve: 2

IMMUNE BOOSTER

Carrots (12 medium)
Oranges (2 large, peeled)
Apple (1 medium)
Beet Root (1 medium)
Lemon (1 small)
Serve: 2

PURPLE PASSION

Apples (4 medium)
Red Cabbage (1/4 head, medium)
Lime (1 medium)
Serve: 1

COOL KALE

Mango (1 medium)

Pineapple (1 cup)

Kale (4 leaf)

Orange (1 small)

Ginger Root (1/2 thump tip)

Serve: 1

POMEGRANATE GREEN

Grapes (2 cups)

Apple (1 medium)

Pomegranate (1 cup)

Celery (4 stalks, medium)

Cucumber (1/2 large)

Spinach (4 cups)

Serve: 2

TURMERIC DELIGHT

Apples (2 medium)

Pears (2 medium)

Celery (3 stalks, large)

Lemons (2 medium, peeled)

Turmeric Root (6 thumb)

Ginger Root (1 thumb tip)

Serve: 2

SWEET POTATO POWER

Carrots (6 medium)

Apples (2 medium)

Zucchini (1 medium)

Orange (1 large)

Sweet Potato (1 medium)

Beet Root (1 medium)

Celery (2 stalks, medium)

Ginger Root (2 thumb tip)

Serve: 2

GIMME A BEET

Pears (3 medium)

Beet Root (1 medium)

Raspberry (1 cup)

Lemon (1 medium)

Serve: 1

CARROT GOODNESS

Apples (2 medium)

Pears (2 medium)

Carrot (4 medium)

Zucchini (1 medium)

Lemon (1 medium)

Ginger Root (2 thumb tip)

Serve: 2

SPICEY SPINACH

Pineapple (3 cups, chunks)

Cucumber (1 large)

Orange (1 large)

Spinach (3 cup)

Ginger Root (2 thumb tip)

Lime (1/2)

Cayenne Pepper (1 dash)

Serve: 2

MORNING GLORY

Apples (2 medium)
Carrots (5 medium)
Orange (1 large)
Sweet Potato (1 medium)
Ginger Root (2 thumb tip)
Turmeric Rood (2 thumb)
Lemon (1/2)
Celery (2 stalks, small)
Serve: 2

15 NATURAL HEALING JUICE RECIPES

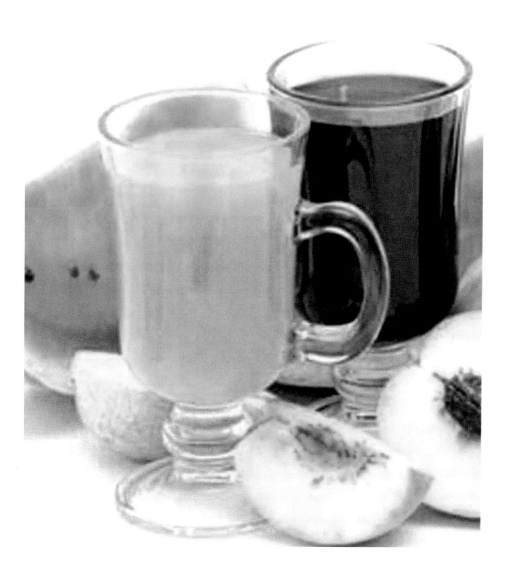

Try juicing these potent combinations if you have any of these issues:

ASTHMA: Carrot, spinach, apple, garlic, lemon

ARTHRITIS: Carrot, cucumber, celery, pineapple

COLD: Carrot, pineapple, ginger, garlic

CONSTIPATION: Carrot, apple, cabbage

DEPRESSION: Carrot, apple, spinach, beet

DIABETES: Carrot, spinach, celery

FATIGUE: Carrots, beet, green apple, lemon, spinach

HANGOVER: Apple, carrot, beet, lemon

HEADACHE: Apple, cucumber, kale, ginger, cucumber, ginger

HIGH BLOOD PRESSURE: Beet, apple, celery, cucumber, ginger

KIDNEY DETOX: Carrot, watermelon, cucumber, ginger

KIDNEY STONE: Orange, apple, watermelon, lemon

MEMORY LOSS: Pomegranate, beets, grape

STRESS: Banana, strawberry, pear

ULCER: Cabbage, carrot, celery

ADD SOME NATURAL ADDITIVES TO YOUR JUICE

Aloe vera: The juice derived from the aloe vera plant can help keep your liver healthy.

Flaxseed: These seed are rich in omega-3 fatty acids, fiber, and protein. Flaxseed also contains lignans, a type of chemical compound that acts as an antioxidant in the body.

Hempseed: The seeds are a more complete protein than milk, meat, and eggs. Hempseed is the seed of the cannabis plant and is rich in fiber and healthy oils.

Psyllium husk: Psyllium is a form of fiber made from the husks of the Plantago ovata plant's seeds. Research show that taking psyllium is beneficial to many parts of the human body, including the heart and the pancreas.

Sea Moss: Consists of 92 minerals of the total 102 mineral that our human body requires; including selenium, calcium, potassium, and magnesium. It helps with thyroid functioning, respiratory issues, weight loss, and energy level.

Wheatgrass: Has anti-cancer benefits and may be part of an effective therapy for ulcerative colitis, indigestion, and overall detoxification.

JUMP START YOUR WEIGHT LOSS JOURNEY

Even when you want to change, old habits sometimes die hard. When most people set out to lose weight it often involves a decision to significantly change their eating habits and to embark on a bold new exercise regimen. In theory this sounds like an effective plan. The reality is that if you set out to workout more, your appetite is likely to go into overload. The key to weight loss is taking in less calories than we burn. To shed a single pound, you need to create a 3,500-calorie deficit: that's a lot of work! Think of it this way: In general, a 150-pound person walking at average speed (from two to three-and-a-half miles per hour) can count on burning about 80 calories a mile. In this example that would equate to burning about 240 calories after walking 3 miles. To put that in perspective, a slice of chocolate cake is approximately 560 calories. Yikes, that's a lot of walking!

Often, we have the faulty belief that since we exercise, we can eat more without gaining weight. The truth is, though, that you'd have to exercise an awful lot just to burn off a small amount of food. A more effective weight loss strategy would be to work on changing our food intake habits, as opposed to moving into the local gym.

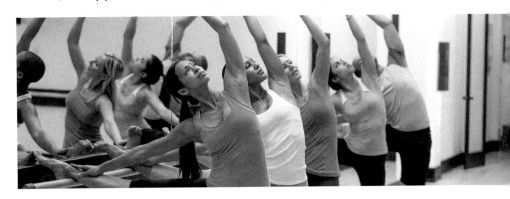

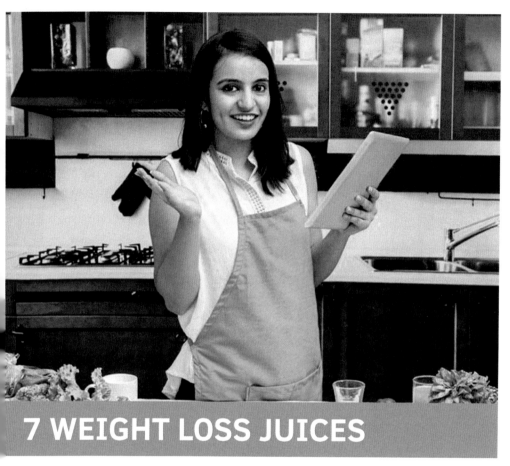

7 WEIGHT LOSS JUICES

1 Carrot Juice

Carrot juice is great for weight loss as carrots are low in calories and full of fiber. Carrot juice is known to increase bile secretion which helps in burning fat thus aiding weight loss.

2 Cucumber Juice

Foods that have high water content are low in calories. Due to its high water and fiber content, cucumber juice fills you up easily.

3 Pomegranate Juice

Pomegranates are rich in antioxidants, polyphenols, and conjugated linolenic acid - all of which help you burn fat and boost your metabolism. Pomegranate juice also helps in suppressing your appetite.

4 Cabbage Juice

Cabbage juice helps in relieving a lot of stomach problems like bloating and indigestion, clears up your digestive tract and helps in quicker elimination of wastes. This aids your weight loss process.

5 Watermelon Juice

This juicy fruit provides only 30 calories per 100 grams and keeps you hydrated. It is rich in amino acid arginine which helps in burning fat.

6 | Orange Juice

Freshly squeezed orange juice could be a healthier, low-calorie alternative to all your fizzy drinks and colas. Orange is a negative calorie fruit which means that it contains fewer calories than what your body requires to burn it.

7 | Pineapple Juice

Pineapple juice is believed to be a great remedy for belly fat. An important enzyme called bromelain which is found in the juice of pineapple helps in metabolizing protein and burns away excess stomach fat. Moreover, bromelain works with other enzymes such as lipase to digest fats and suppress your appetite. Just like oranges, pineapple is also a catabolic food which means that your body spends more calories to burn the fruit than it contains.

JUICE CLEANSE

Whether you are planning to do a 3-day, 7-day, 14-day, or even 30-day juice cleanse, preparation is absolutely, positively the key to the success you deserve.

A juice cleanse is an effective way to ensure you get the fruits and vegetables you need and begin feeding your body the nutrients required to stimulate weight loss and ensure you keep the weight off. After all, losing the weight is only valuable to you if you keep it off, right?

Most of us are creatures of habit. We buy the same foods from the same grocery store, prepare the same recipes over and over, and live within our own familiar routines. But if you're serious about eating more healthfully and losing weight, you're going to need to learn how to shake it up, change those bad eating habits, and start thinking differently about your diet and lifestyle.

The problem is that we get so comfortable in our ways that it is hard to give up those old habits and create a healthier regimen.

Over time, habits become automatic, learned behaviors, and these are stronger than the new habits you are trying to incorporate into your life.

Think a bit about the changes you'd like to make to your diet and write them down if you are willing to commit to them. Then, gradually incorporate these new habits one at a time, slowly. Before you know it, you will be eating more healthfully and losing weight.

Over time, your preferences will change and the cravings for those "bad-for-you" foods will fade away.

Benefits of Juice Cleanse:

Appetite reduction

Elimination of food triggers

Improve your energy

Cell rehydration

Reduction of inflammation

Gentle detox

Rejuvenate your liver

Lose weight

Alkalize your body

Sleep better

Lose belly fat

JUICE CLEANSE QUESTIONS AND ANSWERS

Q. Can I work out during my juice cleanse?

A. Yes. Light or moderate exercise is fine during the cleanse.

Q. How much juice should I drink daily?

A. Strive to drink 72 oz – 96 oz per day of vegetable-based juice daily.

Q. How much weight can I expect to lose during the cleanse?

A. You may lose up to 1lb per day.

Q. How do I break my cleanse?

A. Once you complete your cleanse, consider eating only raw foods for at least 3 days before reintroducing cooked foods to your system.

Q. Can I drink coffee or alcohol during cleanse?

A. Avoid caffeine and alcohol while doing you're cleanse. The toxins contained in both coffee and alcohol can impair liver and kidney function, which may prevent your body being able to cleanse itself naturally. You can drink herbal tea during your cleanse.

Q. What side effects can I expect during my juice cleanse?

A. During the first few days you may experience diarrhea, dizziness, headaches, hunger, or nausea which will normally subside after a few days.

Q. How much water should I consume daily?

A. During your juice cleanse strive to drink 1 gallon of water per day. This will help to flush out toxins and keep you feeling full.

Q. Do I need to take supplements while I am juicing?

A. No. Supplements are used when you are not getting enough nutrients from your diet. Juicing a variety of fruits and vegetables will flood your body with nutrients.

NUTRITIONAL INFORMATION FOR FRUITS

SERVING SIZE = 100G

Food	Calories	Protein	Carbs	Fat	Fiber
Apple	50	0.26	13.81	0.17	2.4
Avocado	160	2.00	8.53	14.60	6.7
Banana	90	1.09	22.84	0.33	2.6
Blackberry	43	1.39	9.61	0.49	5.3
Blueberry	57	0.74	14.49	0.33	2.4
Cantaloupe	34	0.84	8.60	0.19	0.9
Grape	69	0.72	18.00	0.16	0.9
Grapefruit	42	0.77	10.70	0.14	1.7
Kiwi	61	1.00	14.66	0.52	3.0
Lemon	29	1.10	9.32	0.30	2.8
Lime	30	1.00	11.00	0.00	3.0
Mango	70	0.50	17.00	0.27	1.8
Melon	30	0.60	7.60	0.15	0.4
Orange	47	0.94	11.75	0.12	2.4
Papaya	39	0.61	9.81	0.14	1.8
Passion Fruit	97	2.20	23.40	0.70	10.4
Peach	39	0.91	9.54	0.25	1.5
Pear	58	0.38	13.81	0.12	3.1
Pineapple	50	0.54	13.52	0.12	1.4
Pomegranate	83	1.67	18.70	1.17	4.0
Raspberry	52	1.20	11.94	0.65	6.5
Strawberry	32	0.67	7.70	0.30	2.0

NUTRITIONAL INFORMATION FOR VEGETABLES

Food	Calories	Protein	Carbs	Fat	Fiber
Beet	45	1.61	9.56	0.17	2.8
Bell Pepper	31	0.99	6.03	0.30	2.1
Cabbage	25	1.30	5.80	0.10	2.5 mg
Carrot	41	0.93	9.58	0.24	2.8
Cauliflower	25	1.92	4.97	0.28	2.0
Celery	16	1.00	3.00	0.00	2.0
Cucumber	15	0.65	3.63	0.11	0.5
Garlic	149	6.00	33.00	0.00	2.0
Ginger	80	2.00	18.00	1.00	2.0
Kale	50	3.30	10.01	0.70	2.0
Mint	44	3.00	8.00	1.00	7.0
Pumpkin	26	1.00	6.50	0.1	0.5
Spinach	23	2.86	3.63	0.39	2.2
Sweet Potato	86	1.60	20.1	0.05	3.0
Tomato	18	0.90	3.90	0.20	1.2
Zucchini	17	1.21	3.11	0.32	1.0

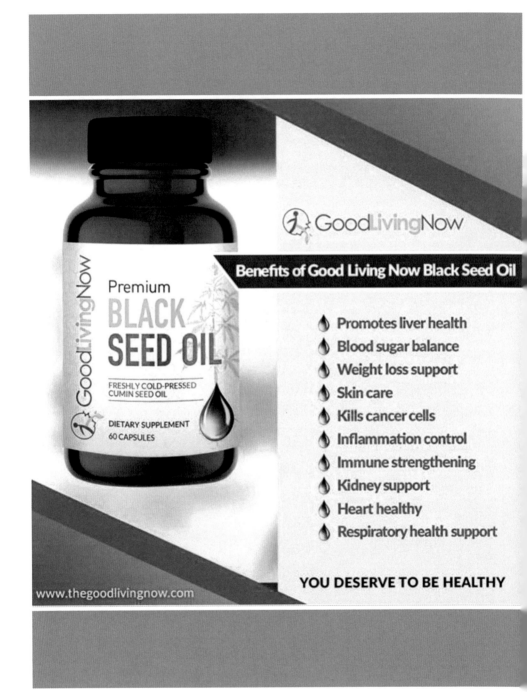

Made in the USA
Middletown, DE
21 August 2024

59560348R00035